Electronic Nicotine Delivery System

Carolyn Ann Vaughan RN

Maritime Home Grown Publishing & Presentations

Dartmouth, Nova Scotia, Canada

Copyright © 2015

Carolyn Ann Vaughan RN

All rights reserved.

ISBN: 978-0-9949443

ISBN: 978-0-9949443-1-3

—

Dedicated to my mother.

Table of Contents

THE BEGINNING

Electronic Nicotine Delivery System

How I became a vaper, and how I inadvertently and even reluctantly gave up a forty-six year pack a day, or better if I was anxious, tobacco habit!

When I began vaping I had absolutely no intention of quitting smoking. In fact, I have been a pro smoker for years. As a Registered Nurse, I have seen a great deal of damage created by those trying to restrict and control tobacco use.

I started seriously smoking tobacco at thirteen. The year was 1963, a package of Export A cigarettes cost about fifty cents a package.

I had actually been caught, by my father, a few years before that, smoking a pilfered cigarette. He decided as a deterrent it might be helpful to have me eat a few cigarettes. Basically, his deterrent plan accomplished me becoming sick to my stomach and better learning how to hide the cigarette packages.

By 1963, I had a part time baby-sitting job, I could buy my own, hide them in the bushes or under my mattress and go my merry way. My father and stepmother were both cigarette smokers therefore couldn't smell me.

The cigarettes hidden under my mattress were raided occasionally so being a creative teenager I hid them in plastic bags in the bushes outside our house.

Tobacco smoking during the 60's and 70's was as common as cell phone use today. People smoked in movie theatres, in restaurants, in hospitals on airplanes.

More than half the adult population smoked tobacco. There was no shame and there was no blame associated with tobacco smoking, in fact, if anything, the act itself was glorified by magazine and television.

I recall when my youngest child was born, smoking in the hospital ward and only extinguishing the cigarette when the baby came from the nursery. For what it's worth, and in case you're curious, all three babies were over eight pounds birth weight, none had allergies, asthma etc., and only one of the three uses tobacco today.

Tobacco use was as common as eating and drinking. I am not sure I can stress the relaxed attitude towards tobacco use. There was no attitude, no guilt, no shame, and no stigma. Tobacco smoking was a non-issue. I suspect anyone under the age of thirty- five would have difficulty believing this, but it is truth. The only taboo I ever recall was, "it is not lady like to smoke on the street" that was it. Then along came social engineering.

By the time I was thirty years old, (1980) I had been smoking about a package a day for fifteen years. It is round about 1980 I decided to give up cigarettes. My reason didn't have anything to do with health, or even finances, it had more to do with the fact I was involved in a choir at the United Church group and many of the members, did not smoke.

Also about this time anti tobacco propaganda and rhetoric was beginning to hit newspaper and magazine articles.

My effort to quit smoking (1980) lasted four years. I gained forty pounds, and was prone to panic attacks. I had a constant pain in the pit of my stomach and underwent numerous tests for suspected ulcers. I frequently craved a cigarette, but by shear will power alone I generally abstained. I often looked forward to any visitors who were smokers. When they visited I would quickly bum a smoke.

I cannot truthfully say my weight gain and my intense anxiety was because I had quit smoking. I don't really know, but I believe it was directly related to giving up tobacco. I also had young children, had returned to school and enrolled in a nursing program so all of these factors could have been the reason for the excessive weight gain and the generalized anxiety I experienced during the four years without tobacco. However, I was convinced my issues were related to lack of nicotine.

What I can say for a fact, was that period of my life was filled with anxiety, and an additional forty pounds.

Socially, tobacco use was becoming more frowned upon but many still smoked and in 1983 when I graduated from nursing school smoking was permitted in the report rooms and on hospital wards.

One of my first run ins with a surgeon was when I suggested he put out his pipe while he visited his patient in one of the bedrooms. I was concerned about the oxygen running in the bedroom. He promptly told me not to be so foolish, "didn't I know oxygen wasn't combustible" and reported me for insubordination to my nursing supervisor the next day.

By 1985, smoking in the bedrooms would change to smoking being permitted in specific sections of the hospital cafeteria.

Somewhere around 1984, a year after I started working as a Registered Nurse, I bummed a cigarette from a colleague, and on my way home from work, I stopped and bought a package, within a week, I once again became a pack a day cigarette smoker.

The fifty-cent pack of smokes I bought at the age of thirteen would become the fifteen-dollar package of smokes I bought at the age of sixty-four.

From the age of thirty-four until I gave up cigarettes at the beginning of this year, I refused to be scolded or shamed into believing I should quit.

I knew how terrible I felt when I wasn't smoking, I knew how anxious I was and I had absolutely no plans whatsoever to give up tobacco. I also was determined not to allow myself to be bullied into giving up tobacco because the government was trying to tax me to death, and I felt a strong sense of camaraderie with fellow smokers who were being increasingly stigmatized by what I considered the mass propaganda machine and questionable methods of population control.

From the beginnings the whole anti smoking tobacco control initiatives stunk to high heavens and personally I believe they still do. And frankly it plain pissed me off and the heavy-handed tactics annoyed me to no end.

Anyone who has known me for the past thirty some years of my nursing career would tell you emphatically, "Carolyn is a smoker with no intentions whatsoever of giving it up." I was irked about the bad press given to those who sold black market cigarettes. A ten year old child could tell you, if smokes on a reservation could be obtained at a quarter of the price of those off reserve then of course your were going to have people buying them at native prices putting a mark up and still making a profit. A government who would tax one segment of society to the tune of 70 percent should hardly be surprised when those not so taxed decide to make a dollar.

PRO TOBACCO ACT

IVIST:

When the tobacco control initiatives became increasingly strident, I became more pro tobacco. I have mountains of letters I wrote to legislators about the damage increasing taxation and tobacco control was dumping on cigarette smokers, especially the poor the elderly and the mental health communities.

I ranted about it to anyone who would listen. I was always the first to offer to take the old lady with her IV pole down to the cafeteria to have her smoke, or to wheel the elderly veteran outdoors when tobacco use became restricted in hospitals.

I think it was round about the year 2000 that nasty pictures on cigarette packs were inflicted on the smoking public, (talk about subliminal advertising) and it was at about this time one of the anti smoking groups started paving the way for a young woman who developed lung cancer to speak to various government bodies about the supposed dangers of second hand smoke.

Hospitals began putting up signs "no smoking" within so many meters of the door.

Privately owned restaurants and clubs were required by law to forbid smoking inside, bingo halls, legions, pubs and taverns and various other gathering places were legislated to not allow smoking inside the facilities. This particular legislation worked further towards keeping the elderly more homebound than not, and was especially annoying to veterans.

And of course along with all the smoking restrictions came the increased taxation always under the guise of preventing kids from smoking.

What happened of course is kids didn't smoke tobacco cigarettes they instead started smoking pot. It was much easier to obtain. Marijuana use skyrocketed while tobacco use decreased. The rise in marijuana use while troubling didn't effect me, I have never been a pot smoker, but I continued to smoke my pack a day of tobacco, out doors of course, in the rain, in the sleet and in the comfort of my car or my home.

I recall an elderly patient restrained in his hospital bed, who quickly became disorganized and confused and because he had been a life long tobacco user, he tried to climb over the rails and ended up breaking his hip. It disgusted me, for want of a cigarette he remained in hospital for months.

I remember an educated woman who told me she lied to her insurance agency about her tobacco use because she did not want to pay higher insurance premiums. I watched young parents sneak cigarettes, thinking they were fooling their children.

I became a smoker's rights activist. I did a tremendous amount of research on nicotine and the tobacco plant and patents on plants etc. I discovered there were huge financial reasons why tobacco was being vilified. Multinationals wanted a patent on the tobacco plant, governments were raking in taxation cash, non – profits were being given grants up the gazoo to stem the tide of tobacco use and every one was winning except the guy on the bottom who derived benefit from nicotine.

In those days you were pretty hard pressed to find any positive attributes of nicotine but I did discover one of the pharmaceutical companies was using nicotine as a benefit to Alzheimer's patients and I saw research supporting nicotine benefits in depression, Parkinson's and Schizophrenia. Eventually this information would become public knowledge.

During the early 90's I worked for a number of years in psychiatry and I noticed just about all psych patients smoked tobacco. They not only smoked tobacco but they were heavy users of tobacco. Common sense would lead one to believe that the patients must have derived see benefits from tobacco.

I knew from personal experience a smoke kept me alert on night shifts and I knew for a fact a smoke steadied my nerves helped me concentrate, similar to a cup of coffee and acted as an appetite suppressant.

I was never, after returning to tobacco in my first year of nursing, one of those folks who made efforts to quit smoking. You never heard me say "I wish I could quit" or "I tried to quit" etc. I simply accepted the fact I was a tobacco smoker and for me the benefits far out weighed any potential problems.

I had grandparents who smoked hand rolled cigarettes and lived well into their eighties.

I was not short of breath, I didn't get frequent colds, and frankly I couldn't see any reason at all to give up what I considered a minor habit, which provided me a lot more benefit than downfall.

As the price of a carton of cigarettes rose, I became more determined to champion the plight of tobacco smokers. And when I started hearing some doctors saying they would not operate on tobacco smokers. It royally pissed me off.

I also became a more dedicated champion of tobacco smokers when a government official told me I should be ashamed of myself (as a nurse) for supporting those who used tobacco. It just plain pissed me off. So I wrote letters and did things like send my complaints to government officials writing on the back of my used cigarette packages. I must have sent over a hundred of these to the Minister of Health.

I would probably still be smoking a pack a day if not for one very important event in my life.

HOW IT CAME TO BE

How I started

I live in Nova Scotia my mother lived in Ontario a distance of about two thousand miles. My mother had been dealing with bowel cancer and in mid January she told me she was checking in to the hospital.

I decided I would travel to Ontario and be with her at the hospital and perhaps provide some support to her and to my stepfather while I was there. My mother had given up tobacco half a lifetime ago, and my stepfather never was a smoker.

I knew I would want to be spending a lot of time at the hospital and when not in the hospital I would be staying with my step dad. Running out doors every few hours in the dead of winter to have a smoke was not my idea of fun, and I really didn't want to stress my mom about my smoking. So I decided I would try vaping.

My young daughter in law said she hadn't smoked for months. She said the vape worked for her. My son had also told me about vaping, said it really did work.

I, like a good tobacco smoker, ignored them both, until mom went in to the hospital.

A few days before my trip to Ontario I went to the vape shop and purchased an Evod. http://www.kangeronline.com/products/evod-starter-kit-with-us-plug?variant=268367366

The above link to the Evod is what my initial purchase of an electronic nicotine delivery system looked like.

I believe mine was maroon in colour. The lad in the vape shop gave me a quick instruction on how to use the Evod. I tried it in the store and although I coughed, I knew immediately it might be possible, it would do what I needed it to do.

I of course told him I had no intention whatsoever of quitting smoking but wanted to use the product while visiting my mom in the hospital. He encouraged me to try flavours at 18 mg nicotine. I of course was adamant I was a tobacco smoker and would only use tobacco flavour so he sold me a tobacco flavour, and just for kicks, because he was being very helpful, I purchased a root beer flavour at 18 mg per ml nicotine.

He explained about the coils and advised me a package of five coils came with the kit and the kit contained two Evods, so I could always have one on the charger.

I brought the contraption home and tried it out for a day before flying to Ontario this was about January 15, of 2015. I packed my suitcase, including my carton of smokes, and set off for Ontario. I checked with the airport to be sure I could fly with my new electronic cigarette. I of course could not use in on the airplane but as soon as I landed, I headed in to the airport bathroom and took a few puffs. The few puffs were sufficient to hold me until I got downstairs to my luggage.

I went directly to the hospital and spent the day with my mother. Occasionally I would excuse myself and go to the bathroom and have a few puffs off the electronic cigarette, and occasionally I would go downstairs out in the cold, off hospital property, to have a real smoke. The first couple of days of use, I noticed I was smoking about three quarters of my usual pack a day of tobacco.

I hadn't yet learned the art of the long slow drag, which is crucial to getting a good supply of nicotine from the electronic cigarette, but I was finding it satisfied my need for nicotine.

It was decided I would stay in the hospital with my mother during the nights. She was alert and appeared to be okay, but my mom was always a person who did not like the nighttime, and I thought perhaps by staying with her at night she would rest easier.

Mom was staying in a ward, and the nurses were kind enough to set me up with a comfy chair for sleeping. I was able to go out and get her ice chips, or rub her back, or just be there with her. Occasionally I would go down to the cafeteria to get her a "real cup of tea"

In the morning my stepfather would arrive to sit with her during the day.

I never told my mother about the electronic cigarette. She would have worried, there was considerable propaganda about electronic cigarettes and I didn't want to put any further stress on her than she already was dealing with. She was sharp as a button and in full control of what she wanted and what she didn't, and although she was critically ill she was a pleasure to be with.

When I went back to her house I would occasionally smoke tobacco cigarettes outside, in the snow, but inside I would use the electronic cigarette. I learned how to change the coil and I learned how to make sure I always kept the spare electronic cigarette charged. I figured I would be in Ontario for months, staying at the hospital at night and sleeping at her home during the day.

MOM'S DEATH

My mom passed away surrounded by family less than a week after I went to Ontario. I don't really know how to describe the death of my mother she died peacefully but for me it was and still is a tremendous loss. I knew it was coming, but I was still not prepared for it. I am grateful I was able to spend those few nights with her. I am grateful she did not seem to be in pain until the very last, but I miss her. I suspect I will always miss her. She was my mother.

Mom died January 21, 2015. She passed away during the worse Canadian winter we have had in a very long time, her visitation was on Feb 1, and her Funeral service was in the middle of a blizzard on Feb 2, 2015. The reason for the long delay between her death and the funeral service was so relatives from Nova Scotia could arrive, also Mom had been actively involved in her church and requested a beloved pastor, preside at her funeral service and when she passed away he was in British Columbia.

During the time of her hospitalization and until her funeral service I continued to use the electronic cigarette, going outdoors in the raging winter to smoke tobacco but using the electronic cigarette inside, either in her guest apartment or in the bathroom.

I didn't tell many people about the electronic cigarette, and the few I did mention it to would often say, "I heard those were as bad for you as real cigarettes."

What I began to notice was the real cigarettes tasted terrible and I often could not finish a whole one, but being a smoker of tobacco for well over 46 years I was reluctant to let an old friend go. So I continued to use both the electronic cigarette and real tobacco. I also began to notice I actually preferred the root beer taste juice to the tobacco taste juice. It surprised me but I went with it. If I wanted a smoke I had a smoke-outside of course, but I found I simply didn't want one that often.

I was smoking about a half a package a day during a time in my life when I was experiencing one of life's most stressful events, the passing of my mother.

One day I decide I would make a trip to a vape shop to see what other equipment might be available and to purchase more nicotine fluid. I chose to purchase 12 mg per ml nicotine instead of the 18mg the lad in Nova Scotia sold me, and I added another flavour to my collection.

I believe it was chocolate mint. I discovered I truly did not like the taste of tobacco and actually purchased another starter kit to give to my brother along with the tobacco flavoured juice,

The shop in Ontario sold me an istick Eleaf, he told me the battery would hold a charge for days, which it will, and that I could adjust the wattage. I didn't know anything about wattage but the Eleaf was a pretty pink and about the size of a nine-volt battery, so I bought it. http://www.istick.org/

He also suggested the nautilus mini. http://www.aspirecig.com/products/tank-series/tank156.html

A glass than made by Aspire, he suggested it was superior to my Evod Kangertech. While I did prefer the Eleaf battery to the Kangertech battery, I couldn't manage to get the nautilaus mini to work properly.

It would gurgle and no matter what I did it seemed to provide a less satisfying vapour. This eventually changed when I learned how to use the nautilus mini.

I recall telling one person about my troubles with the nautilaus mini and he suggested perhaps I had a counterfeit product. Apparently sales of the mini were so popular companies were counterfeiting them to keep up with demand.

BACK HOME AGAIN

Mid February, in the middle of the worst blizzard Atlantic Canada had seen in years my hubby and I returned from Ontario. I recall standing at the airport in the bus shelter waiting for a bus to take us to our home. I was sorrowful, exhausted and stressed out. There was no way I would be able to light up a smoke, but I had no problem taking a puff off my electronic cigarette, and it was sufficient to settle my anxieties.

The next couple of weeks would determine whether or not I would toss the electronic cigarette in a drawer and go back to my pack a day of tobacco.

I was on my home turf, still hurting from the passing of my mother and returning to a job as a nurse on a forensic psychiatric unit.

What I was fast discovering is that no matter how I tried to kid myself, I actually did not enjoy the tobacco smokes. They tasted like ashtrays and although I was forcing myself to smoke about five a day, I was not enjoying them at all. I would take a few drags off the tobacco cigarette and then put it out. I also noticed I could often times go on my work break and just use the electronic cigarette and not have any tobacco at all. It was a major surprise to me.

I also became aware that a fair number of other nurses and a doctor were using electronic cigarettes.

At the same time, there were massive publicity articles in newspapers etc., citing the evils of the electronic cigarette, listing it with illegal drug use, or unmentionable health problems, blah blah, blah.

I was in a bit of a pickle I was truly disliking my tobacco smokes and favouring my electronic vapour. My hubby who had given up tobacco a few years previously was happy to share the car with me and my house, clothes and hands smelled better. I was accustomed to putting out at least a hundred dollars a week for smokes. I was now putting out twenty dollars a week for nicotine liquid.

The only health effect I could notice was a bit of a dry throat, which went away if I drank a little more water. But I still hadn't found a flavour I could tolerate all day long, one I truly loved.

Fruit juice flavours didn't do much for me, and I no longer liked chocolate mint.

Finally I went back to the vape shop and selected "Vader Puddin" by Maple Leaf Vapes.

MARCH 1ˢᵗ I QUIT

By the end of February, about six weeks after I started using the electronic nicotine delivery system. I was down to half a tobacco butt a day and on March 1st, 2015 I decided to stop fighting with myself, forcing myself to have a tobacco cigarette and just quit.

I loved my "Vader Pudding" and on top of that it was a mixture of 40 % USP Vegetable Glycerine and 60% USP Propylene Glycol.

Most of the other juices I had tried were 30% USP Vegetable Glycerine and 70 % USP Propylene Glycol. The difference made for a smoother vape, and tasted like toffee. I bought an 18 mg nicotine bottle and a 12 mg nicotine bottle and happily vaped my way through about six bottles of the stuff.

My nicotine delivery system liquid was costing me about twenty-five dollars a week compared to over a hundred dollars a week for tobacco.

I of course told myself I could have a tobacco cigarette anytime I wanted one but why in Gods name would I want something, which tasted like sh....

I would have been in heaven except, one day I went to the vape shop for my usual weekly bottle of Vader Puddin and the lad was sold out.

Eeks, not good! I finally found a bit of a replacement for the Vader Puddin, but it was more expensive.

It dawned on me I was becoming dependent on the manufacturer always having a taste and solution I preferred.

Also, there was a lot of political talk about taxing the electronic cigarette supplies and vape shops would no longer be permitted to let you sample the flavours.

I started doing more research and discovered seventy percent of the cost of a carton of tobacco went toward Government taxes. Tobacco was/and is a huge cash cow for both federal and provincial governments.

http://www.smokefree.ca/factsheets/pdf/totaltax.pdf

I of course knew hospitals dished out nicotine replacements such as gum and patches by the bucket load.

Very few patients I had ever met actually quit smoking using the gum or the patch but it was considered okay to dispense in the hospital BUT something actually working, the electronic cigarette with liquid nicotine, was not supported or encouraged in fact was denigrated and scorned by numerous pundits. Hospital administration was a strong naysayer.

I made efforts at the place where I worked to see if I could introduce our patients to an electronic nicotine delivery system. I was told I could not, the same way I was told we could not put a bench outdoors, half way up the hill for the tobacco smokers to use-"it might encourage them to smoke on hospital property."

Instead, those who used tobacco, about eighty percent of our inpatients, were required to leave hospital property and walk about a quarter mile up a steep hill to smoke. Leaving hospital property to smoke caused tremendous hardships to the patients, caused elderly people to slip and fall on the ice and put both themselves and others at extreme risk, but that is another story.

During the time I was finding the electronic nicotine delivery system to be the most effective stop smoking program I had ever encountered, I started to foresee a number of places where I could be held captive to a system run by multinational organizations and groups having agendas and political hoopla which would be counterproductive to me.

Pharmaceutical companies of course are anti ecig, they are okay with nicotine, in fact they have put much effort towards showing the benefits of nicotine as a mild anti depressants, a help with Alzheimer's, Parkinson's, and Schizophrenia, but of course the pharmaceutical conglomerates want the ability to control the electronic cigarette supply.

The other group who is anti electronic cigarette (until they can tax it to the hilt like tobacco cigarettes) is the government. Also involved in the rag tag mess of people who have been milking the tobacco propaganda train for years, the non profit groups, are anti electronic nicotine delivery system. For years they have made a fortune scaring the daylights out of tobacco users and their families taking handouts from the tobacco companies, the Government and the pharmaceutical companies. They don't really want anyone to give up tobacco, not really.

So what could I do? I am fully aware of the benefits of nicotine to me, and I have no intention (at least not in the foreseeable future) of giving up nicotine.

Manufacturers of liquid nicotine and suppliers of the electronic cigarette are vulnerable to laws and damning public opinion. I started more research and found ECF the electronic cigarette forum to be a reliable and useful source of information.

https://www.e-cigarette-forum.com/forum/

Another site I considered helpful regarding information on equipment was Phil Busardos site "Taste Your Juice"

http://www.tasteyourjuice.com/

My final conclusion was, unless I wished to be caught in the same price trap I had seen tobacco go through over the years I would need to take matters into my own hands and provide my own control of my nicotine use.

I knew I would have to find a way to protect myself from the laws, the potential for increased taxation and the possibility of a complete ban on electronic cigarette supplies.

I learned how to make my own coils and I read about how to make my own juice. I currently make my own nicotine juice, flavour it myself and decide what strength nicotine I will use.

I am Canadian, we have quirky laws in Canada regarding nicotine liquid, Health Canada does not currently champion the electronic nicotine delivery system, but who knows now that we are considering legalizing marijuana perhaps they shall revisit the issue. I have a hard time understanding how we can legalize marijuana, yet denigrate and put roadblocks in front of nicotine use. It is like comparing coffee to whiskey.

It is expensive for Canadian suppliers to purchase nicotine liquid and as far as I know they are not yet producing liquid nicotine in Canada, though this too may change.

Given all the possible roadblocks I decided I would purchase a liter of liquid nicotine from the United States. By spending some time on the electronic cigarette forum I realized there were numerous suppliers, but the one I chose was: My Freedom Smokes:

https://www.myfreedomsmokes.com/liquid-nicotine-eliquid-vapes-unflavored.html

The cost for one liter of 100 mg per ml liquid nicotine was ninety dollars tax, exchanges and delivery included. I was informed by the owner of My Freedom Smokes that there was a possibility Canadian Customs would not deliver the liter of liquid and would in fact return it to the manufacturer.

I had my plan, if customs refused to deliver the liquid nicotine I was prepared to make a royal stink. I come from a generation of sign carrying, civil rights activists and was prepared to do whatever it took to bring this situation to public scrutiny.

Sadly to say I didn't get the opportunity to confront the powers that be. The liter of nicotine liquid I ordered from the states was delivered without incident, too bad really because I would have enjoyed the challenge.

The liter of nicotine liquid, which cost me ninety dollars is sufficient to allow me to make five hundred 25 ml bottles of nicotine juice, basically enough juice to last me about ten years give or take. Or in other words at todays price for store bought nicotine juice about ten thousand dollars worth of juice.

Or put a different way, with my ninety dollar bottle of 100 mg per ml nicotine liquid I can make enough 8 mg per ml juice to prevent me paying 52 thousand dollars for tobacco cigarettes during the next ten years (I would easily smoke a carton of cigarettes each and every week and a carton of cigarettes is currently selling for over one hundred dollars.) And by using my own nicotine liquid I would not be contributing over 36 thousand dollars in tobacco tax.

Just looking at what I have written and I am still astounded I have escaped. I am writing this book because I am hoping you too will escape. I also believe it is important to understand the powerful forces that wish to frightened you about the electronic nicotine delivery system.

If you are still smoking tobacco today, you are quite likely a person who benefits from nicotine. I stay this because since about 1990, you have been inundated with the dangers of cigarette smoke have been subject to mass propaganda and been shamed and your tobacco smoke has been blamed for just about every evil known to man.

You have been guilted, taxed beyond measure, and segregated. Meanwhile the profiteers (and the Government is most certainly one of the profiteers) have done everything in their power to keep you there.

The government wants to keep you there, the tobacco company wants to keep you there, the pharmaceutical company wants to keep you there and believe it or not so does the anti tobacco group want to keep you there. Isn't it perhaps time you took back your own control?

Some will say, ah but Carolyn what about the health risks. Yes, what about them? I don't know. I know my liquid contains four ingredients, Nicotine, propylene glycol, vegetable glycerine and a drop of flavouring. Now that I make my own juice, I use only a small amount of flavouring.

I know I started out nine months ago using 18 mg per ml nicotine I now use 8 mg per ml nicotine. (I still vape about 25 ml per week) I have absolutely no cravings for tobacco at all. Let me repeat that, I have absolutely no cravings for tobacco at all; in fact I don't even use tobacco-flavoured juice. I don't like the taste.

I have absolutely no cough. I smell nice. I don't have to worry about burning ashes. I no longer have to be concerned about the government increasing the taxes on supplies, or banning the electronic nicotine delivery system. I know how to make a simple coil if I need to, I know how to store my nicotine fluid and I know how to care for my battery.

I know my tobacco cigarette contains thousands of chemicals, which I no longer ingest. I know I spend five hundred dollars less from my pension cheque each month on a nicotine supplement.

I know I now have control over how much nicotine I use and the strength I use. I use a free online juice calculator:

http://www.steam-engine.org/juice.asp

I do not make ejuice for anyone else, but considering the extreme markup I can understand why some would.

When my 1000 ml bottle arrived, I carefully transferred it to four dark brown glass bottles, labeled it, wrapped it in newspaper and stored it in the fridge. I make my juice every two weeks. I usually make two 25 ml bottles of juice at a time, enough to last me two weeks. I have two Eleaf batteries, one pink and one blue.

I am very careful with my nicotine liquid in high doses it is very toxic so I use gloves when I am mixing it. I also use a five ml syringe for accuracy. I vary my flavouring, but generally use, cotton candy, cappuccino, Kahlua, brandy, coconut, blueberry, or strawberry. A use only few drops of flavour in each bottle. I haven't purchased "store bought" juice for the past six months. My weekly nicotine delivery system costs me about the same price as a cup of coffee.

If, and I say if, I were to experience a strong craving for a tobacco cigarette, or even a mild craving for a tobacco cigarette I would mix up a bottle of juice using 12 mg per ml nicotine and use that for a bit.

So far I have experienced absolutely no cravings at all. I may at some point in the future decrease the amount of nicotine, if I do decide to do this, I would make one bottle at 8 mg nicotine per ml and the other at 4 mg per ml and expect that I would use the electronic vaporizer a little more frequently at the lower nicotine dosage until my body becomes accustomed to the lower dosage.

I now have control, and that my friends continues to amaze me.

If you choose to try the electronic nicotine delivery system, please do your research. Read everything you can about how to use the equipment, how to clean it how to keep your battery charged, how to always have a spare, fully charged battery on hand.

I had absolutely no intention of quitting cigarettes when I started this whole experiment, and I frequently told myself I would only continue with the electronic vapour until I no longer found it workable or satisfying, but I have found it to be an incredibly easy process.

After forty-six years of smoking a daily package of cigarettes I no longer smoke tobacco and since March 1st, I have saved over thirty six hundred dollars of which twenty-five hundred would have gone to the government in taxes.

I have heard of some folks who were determined to quit smoking that picked up a starter set and never had another tobacco cigarette.

I have heard of others who have tried the kind without nicotine who have failed miserably. I have heard of folks who have started but, listened to the naysayers and gave up "because it isn't proven safe"

I say it works and for me, it is the only thing that has, and I never even intended to quit!

http://discovermagazine.com/2014/march/13-nicotine-fix

https://en.wikipedia.org/wiki/Nicotine

https://en.wikipedia.org/wiki/Electronic_cigarette

I have included links in this booklet for your use, they are not the only links on the electronic cigarette subject and there are numerous suppliers of both equipment and juice, the inks I have provided are the ones I used.

I have made the best choice for me of this I am certain. You need to decide for yourself if it is a choice you wish to make.

The World Health Organization does not yet support any electronic nicotine delivery system.

ABOUT THE AUTHOR

Carolyn Ann Vaughan is a retired Registered Nurse. This is her second book. She has worked as a nurse in three provinces, on a First Nations Reserve and at a hospice in one American State. Throughout her nursing career she has written for publication and has had articles published in the East Coast Gardener, The Dartmouth Laker and The National Review of Medicine. She currently lives in Dartmouth, with her husband and three goldfish. She enjoys reading, gardening, guitar, her family and her church. She is currently at work on her first full-length thriller, "Life in the Trenches" due to be released in the spring of 2016.

<<<<>>>

www.ingramcontent.com/pod-product-compliance
Lightning Source LLC
Chambersburg PA
CBHW071343290326
41933CB00040B/2159